Fuzzy Buzzy Groups for Children with Developmental and Sensory Processing Difficulties

Fuzzy Buzzy Groups for Children with Developmental and Sensory Processing Difficulties

A Step-by-Step Resource

Fiona Brownlee and Lindsay Munro

Illustrated by: Aisling Nolan

Jessica Kingsley Publishers
London and Philadelphia

First published in 2010
by Jessica Kingsley Publishers
116 Pentonville Road
London N1 9JB, UK
and
400 Market Street, Suite 400
Philadelphia, PA 19106, USA

www.jkp.com

Library of Congress Cataloging in Publication Data

Brownlee, Fiona.
  Fuzzy buzzy groups for children with developmental and sensory processing difficulties : a step-by-step resource / Fiona Brownlee and Lindsay Munro ; illustrated by Aisling Nolan.
       p. cm.
  Includes bibliographical references.
  ISBN 978-1-84310-966-2 (pb : alk. paper) 1. Developmentally disabled children--Education. I. Munro, Lindsay. II. Title.
  LC4661.B727 2009
  371.92--dc22
                                                                         2009009955

British Library Cataloguing in Publication Data
A CIP catalogue record for this book is available from the British Library

ISBN 978 1 84310 966 2

Printed and bound in Great Britain by
Athenaeum Press, Gateshead, Tyne and Wear

Contents

About the Authors   8

Preface   9

Acknowledgements   11

1   **Introduction**   13

     What is a Fuzzy Buzzy Group?   13

     Who can run a Fuzzy Buzzy Group?   15

     Where can you run a Fuzzy Buzzy Group?   15

     Positive feedback   15

     Conclusion   16

2   **How the Fuzzy Buzzy Group Works**   18

     Important aspects of the group   18

     What contribution can a Fuzzy Buzzy Group make to a child's

     development and skills?   19

     Compatibility with educational curriculums   20

3   **What is Sensory Processing?**   22

     What are our senses?   22

     Why are these senses important?   26

     Sensory processing difficulties in children   27

     Encouraging appropriate responses   29

     Behaviour   29

4   **Child Development**   30

     Children's developmental stages   31

     What is developmental delay?   33

     Developmental age versus developmental stage   34

     Developmental delay and typical characteristics   35

     Physical or learning disabilities   35

5 How to Select Appropriate Children. 36

  Children diagnosed with sensory processing difficulties 36

  Behaviours that suggest a child will benefit from a
  Fuzzy Buzzy Group 38

  Children unsuitable to attend a Fuzzy Buzzy Group 39

  Involving parents 39

6 Running the Group. 41

  Preparing to run the group 41

  Laying out the room for a Fuzzy Buzzy Group 42

  Selecting sensory themes. 44

  Final preparations before you run the session. 45

7 Now You Can Begin 46

  Step 1 Hello. 46

  Step 2 Sensory bags 47

  Step 3 Drink preparation 48

  Step 4 Teddies go to hide 49

  Step 5 Sensory path 50

  Step 6 Snack time. 51

  Step 7 Goodbye. 52

  General tips for the session leader 53

  General tips for adults involved in running a session. 53

  Watching out for over-stimulation. 54

8 Finding Sensory Materials 55

  Resources list: the sensory bags. 56

  Resources list: the tunnel and the sensory path 59

  Sensory item recipes 60

9 Choosing Sensory Food and Drink 62

  Equipment for preparing the food and drink 62

  Food suggestions 62

  Drink suggestions. 63

  Using the liquidizer 64

10 Helpful Resources. **65**

Books. 65

Specialist sensory suppliers 66

Useful Handouts, Templates and Forms

Consent Form

What is Sensory Processing?

Confirmation Letter

Fuzzy Buzzy Song (CD track 1)

All Together Now (CD track 2)

Let Us Have a Look (CD track 3)

Socks and Shoes (CD track 4)

Goodbye (CD track 5)

Feeding Checklist

Sensory/Behaviour Form

Evaluation Form

Teddy Bear Badge and Sticker Templates

General Tips for Adults Involved in Running a Session

Fuzzy Buzzy Session Planner

About the Authors

Fiona Brownlee, Dip. COT, BSc in Occupational Therapy, COSCA Certificate in Counselling. Fiona qualified as an occupational therapist (OT) in Edinburgh in 1969. Since then, she has worked in many fields, including psychiatry, orthopaedics, stroke rehabilitation and, since 1989, in paediatrics. In 1992 Fiona worked for four months in Romanian orphanages and has returned for follow-up visits. With her commitment to supporting students on placement, Fiona is a visiting lecturer at university and college level.

Fiona's particular interest lies in the early years and she has completed Signalong, Hanen and Solihull training, among many other courses which she has undertaken. Fiona is trained in counselling and in 1997, upgraded her Dip. COT to a BSc. She has been based in the City of Edinburgh's Children and Families Department since 1998, working as a peripatetic OT, supporting children, parents and staff in the city's child and family centres.

Lindsay Munro, BSc in Occupational Therapy. Since her graduation from Queen Margaret University, Edinburgh, in 2003, Lindsay began working as a paediatric occupational therapist with the Children and Families Department in Edinburgh, supporting children and staff in the child and family centres and at home. Lindsay has recently taken up a new post as a senior paediatric occupational therapist, working in the community with children and young people aged 0–18, who have varying conditions. Lindsay has attended various training courses, which have improved her expertise in working with children experiencing physical, developmental and sensory processing difficulties. She regularly attends many professional interest groups relating to her practice and has qualified as a practice placement educator.

Lindsay provides frequent in-service courses for allied health professionals, teachers, nursery nurses and parents and is a committee member of East Central Scotland College of Occupational Therapists (Specialist Section, Children, Young People and Families), which involves organizing study events, attending committee and national executive meetings and organizing the national annual conference. In 2006, Lindsay carried out voluntary work in Romania, working in an orphanage as a paediatric occupational therapist.

Preface

As paediatric occupational therapists, we have worked with many children exhibiting a wide range of sensory and cognitive difficulties. It is evident that these children benefit from structure, predictability and routine, yet we could find very little, in the literature and support materials available, which provided appropriate advice, methods and strategies for working with this client group. As we are constantly trying to develop and improve our therapy service, in 2003 we decided to carry out a study into parental satisfaction with our occupational therapy service provision.

Parents identified four main areas as being most important to their child's therapy:

- Children should receive more direct intervention.

- Children should be encouraged to mix with other children experiencing similar difficulties.

- Parents should receive more information regarding developmental and sensory issues.

- Parents should be given more opportunity to meet other parents of children experiencing similar difficulties.

Having identified the needs of the parents and found no suitable programmes currently available, we devised the Fuzzy Buzzy Group programme. It was implemented, monitored and evaluated with two independent groups on separate occasions and using both standardized and non-standardized assessments. Not only were the parents delighted with the programme, but also the nursery staff were very enthusiastic. Statistically significant improvements were measured in the children's sensory processing and behaviour. The results of this research were extremely positive and have been published in the College of Occupational Therapists, Specialist Section, Children, Young People and Families Journal (Brownlee and Munro 2005, 2006).

Sensory processing difficulties (SPD) negatively affect children's ability to benefit from the education they receive and can be considered as an 'additional support need'. Given the lack of materials to support children with SPD in mainstream settings, we have designed the programme to support the inclusion of children with additional support needs.

We appreciate that there are different terminologies used for describing sensory processing difficulties, such as 'sensory integration' or 'sensory modulation'. However, for the purpose of this book, we shall use the term 'sensory processing difficulties' throughout.

References

Brownlee, F. and Munro, L. (2005) 'Service review: Evaluation of parents' satisfaction with occupational therapy provided in the City of Edinburgh's child and family centres.' *National Association of Paediatric Occupational Therapy Journal 9*, 1, 11–15.

Brownlee, F. and Munro, L. (2006) 'A pilot study of parental involvement in an occupational therapy group for children with sensory difficulties.' College of Occupational Therapists, Specialist Section, *Children, Young People and Families Journal 10*, 3, 9–14.

Acknowledgements

Thanks to: Gael Munro, MEd, Chartered Teacher, who read through the text carefully and offered constructive amendments from a teacher's perspective; Katie Evans, Eileen Muirhead, Fiona Douglas, Julie Ireland and Nicola Dickson (nursery officers from child and family centres, City of Edinburgh Council); Carrie Evans, occupational therapy student, Queen Margaret University, Edinburgh, who carried out the standardized assessments pre and post groups; Aisling Nolan, BSc Hons Art Therapist, for her illustrations; Eric Wood, BA, PGCE (FE) for his musical arrangements, vocals, fiddle and banjo.

Lastly, we would like to offer a special thanks to all the parents and children who have participated in our research and Fuzzy Buzzy Groups.

1
Introduction

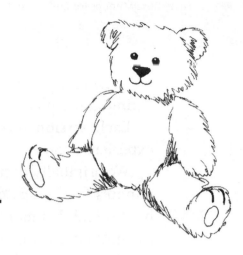

What is a Fuzzy Buzzy Group?

This resource is designed for adults working with young children who are struggling with daily activities and may be avoiding everyday senses and experiences.

Children with sensory processing difficulties are sometimes seen as 'loners' or 'drifters' who find it difficult to settle to any one activity and who may find it difficult to make friends or play interactively with other children. Conversely, they can be hyperactive and oversensitive to the world around them and have difficulty with social skills, which can also isolate them from their peers. They are commonly seen to have behavioural problems which often arise from the difficulties they have in processing sensory experiences.

We have designed this programme to be a practical resource for exploring sensory experiences that is fun, themed based and music led, and which is structured across eight sessions. Accompanying each session are songs, which are intended to be simple, catchy and important in helping the child to refocus and be aware that an activity is about to happen. It is amazing how quickly children learn routines through repetitive tunes. The music and songs are available on the CD provided and the lyrics are provided in the Handouts section.

Central to the Fuzzy Buzzy Group programme is the theme of a 'teddy bears' picnic'. At each session, children bring their own teddy bear (or favourite fuzzy soft toy) and participate in sensory activities before following a 'sensory path' to a hidden picnic spot, where their teddy bear has been left sitting around the picnic table by one of the adults. Towards the end of the session, each child follows the path to find their teddy bear, who will be sitting at the picnic table waiting for them at the end of their journey.

Each session follows a similar format, but explores different sensory experiences on each occasion.

We originally designed each session to run for around an hour and fifteen minutes for groups of up to eight children (as turn-taking is involved, we have found that more than eight tends to become difficult). Ideally, the adult to child ratio is one to one. Sometimes parents can be enlisted to assist, but this is not essential.

The programme is designed to be cost-effective, as many of the items required can be obtained free or at low cost, or can be reused again and again.

Please feel free to adapt this content as required according to your own needs and the children's levels of concentration. For example, you may opt to leave out the food element of the 'snack time' section of the programme if finances are limited.

We found that children with a functioning developmental age of between two and five years benefit most from the programme. Some children who are older but who have developmental delay may also enjoy the programme and not find it childish (for example, a six-year-old who is functioning as a three-year-old). The activities are designed to be inclusive, so while they are particularly useful for children with SPDs, they can also be fun for any child!

As children learn through repetition, it is recommended that the programme is run at regular intervals. We have found it particularly effective over the course of eight weeks. However, it is equally feasible to run the programme on a daily basis, or even dipping in to run a session when a window of opportunity presents itself.

We have run the programme with and without parental involvement on a weekly and daily basis. All groups have been extremely successful and have given excellent results.

The programme requires participating children to engage with messy play activities, so parents should be asked to supply the child with an additional set of clothes to change into at the end.

Practitioners are now expected to evidence their practice in order to justify the intervention they carry out with a child, and so we have provided a photocopiable Evaluation Form which should be completed at the end of the programme and can be used to monitor and assess changes in the children.

Who can run a Fuzzy Buzzy Group?

While we are qualified occupational therapists, you do not need to possess the same qualification in order to run a Fuzzy Buzzy Group. We have devised this programme in a way that can be used by a wide range of professionals, including early years practitioners, teachers, teaching assistants and family respite carers.

The group can be run by any interested member of staff who is willing to develop a greater understanding of sensory processing difficulties and to follow the guidelines provided in this resource. Whoever does run the group must be willing to help all children participate to the best of their ability and minimize the effects of the differences in children's abilities.

It is important that parental consent is sought before a child attends this group. Parents should also be encouraged by staff members to come along and help with running the group if they wish.

Where can you run a Fuzzy Buzzy Group?

The simplicity of the programme means that it can be run in a wide range of settings. While the programme may be carried out in a nursery or primary school setting, community centres or clubs are also suitable, provided there is a reasonably sized room to accommodate the children (and any adults in attendance). We recommend that the group is carried out indoors in order to prevent the children having to cope with additional external stimuli, such as cars, planes or unknown voices.

Positive feedback

Here is some of the positive feedback we have received from people who have already taken part in running Fuzzy Buzzy Groups:

Katie Evans (Nursery Nurse, Child and Family Centre):
I found that the Fuzzy Buzzy Group was very interesting and beneficial to all who attended. I feel that having been part of the programme and having read the resource I am now confident enough to run the programme independently without the assistance

of an occupational therapist. This programme has been needed for a long time.

Nicola Dickson (Nursery Nurse, Child and Family Centre):

Initially, the children were unfamiliar with the routine and struggled to cope with what was expected of them. However, this developed over the course of the eight weeks and the children became less apprehensive and joined in nearly all of the sensory activities.

Julie Ireland (Nursery Nurse, Child and Family Centre):

The programme was well organized, planned and resourced and when I was involved in running it I felt confident and relaxed.

Gael Munro (MEd, Chartered Teacher):

This book offers excellent practical support and ideas for teachers to build on. I would heartily recommend it to colleagues.

Parent:

It was great to observe my child and be pointed in the right direction. I liked being involved in therapy and I now have a greater understanding of why my child behaves the way he does. I found it supportive being amongst other parents who had children with similar difficulties.

Susan Moore (Occupational Therapy Student):

All the children selected appeared to benefit from the routine and predictability of the group. By the end of the programme their compliance has improved and their interaction with their peers was noticeably better. It was a joy to watch.

Conclusion

To summarize, Fuzzy Buzzy Groups

- are suitable for a wide range of people working with children
- address the issues that concern parents of children with sensory processing difficulties in a relaxed, fun and easy-to-follow manner
- help children who experience sensory processing difficulties to tolerate the environmental stimulation to which they are exposed in everyday life

- can help children with the behavioural problems that often accompany sensory processing difficulties

- are time-effective and cost-effective

- support the inclusion of children in mainstream settings, and can be run for children with, or without, additional support needs

- help to develop children's overall development through a routine-based, structured programme.

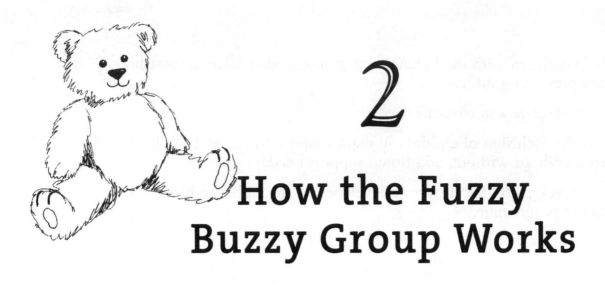

2

How the Fuzzy Buzzy Group Works

Important aspects of the group

The catchy name of 'Fuzzy Buzzy Group' and the theme of a teddy bear's picnic are both intended to be memorable for the children taking part. An essential feature of the group is that it must be fun and motivational. Catchy names, tunes and routines all contribute to the success of the group, as it reminds the children where they are going and what is about to happen. The familiar songs and music act as signifiers to prepare for the next activity.

The children selected to participate in the programme have an important contribution to make, as the activities encourage them to develop a rapport with one another. There is no competitive element within this programme, thus helping to develop a feeling of equality and togetherness. This, along with the distribution of 'teddy bear' badges at the end of each session, help to promote group identity.

A key feature of the programme is that it follows a predictable and familiar routine each time. It is imperative that the format remains exactly the same each week by following the seven steps:

1. Hello

2. Sensory bags (each child is given a sensory bag containing an item to explore)

3. Drink preparation (each child prepares a 'sensory drink' to consume later, at snack time)

4. Teddies go to hide (when the teddy bear is taken away from the child and moved to a seat in the hidden picnic area)

5. Sensory path (when the children journey along the sensory path to join their teddies in the picnic area, see p.50)

6. Snack time (where the picnic takes place – the prepared drink is consumed, with a snack)

7. Goodbye.

The only feature of the seven steps that changes from one session to the next is the nature of the the sensory experience: which items are placed in the sensory bags, what material is used on the sensory path, and what food and drink is consumed. The rigid structure provides children with a predictable routine that enables them to feel more confident about exploring different sensory experiences.

The children who particularly benefit from attending this group often require repetition in order to learn and consolidate new skills. Therefore, good planning and organization by the adults is essential.

We have provided a Feeding Checklist and a Sensory/Behaviour Form to be completed after each session (see Handouts section). These are designed to keep a record of the child's responses to the senses introduced and they can be analysed at a later date to see if there are any trends that develop or if the child appears to be tolerating a particular sense more as the sessions continue. For example, children may react to a particular sensation by turning away, crying, or wiping their hands on their clothes or on the floor, but in subsequent sessions, they may ask for more food, or show delight and enthusiasm for the sensory item that week.

What contribution can a Fuzzy Buzzy Group make to a child's development and skills?

Social skills

Participation in group work enables children to observe and interact with their peers. It provides a group identity and a common bond, thus reassuring the adults and children that they are not the only ones who are experiencing such difficulties. Friendships can be established and social skills reinforced.

Turn-taking

Many children find it difficult to wait, share toys and/or take turns. By using repetition, example and praise, they begin to learn these skills, such as taking turns to walk along the path or press the switch, waiting to receive their sensory bag and sharing their sensory items.

Listening skills

The activities also help to develop the children's listening skills.

Self-esteem

By learning new skills and feeling more confident, the children's self-esteem can improve.

Sequencing

The rigid structure of group routines assists children to develop their ability to sequence tasks.

Object permanence

Part of the routine involves the teddies going away and being found again. While this might initially cause some distress, the children soon learn that although they cannot see their teddy, it has not gone forever. This is called object permanence.

Compatibility with educational curriculums

Although the original concept of the Fuzzy Buzzy Group was to address sensory processing difficulties and associated challenging behaviour in children, it also develops other developmental skills: there are many children who would benefit from this programme.

The eight session programme is designed to promote continuity and consolidation of learning reflecting the areas listed below, but the basic structure of the programme could be adapted to suit the needs of the children or a particular establishment or curriculum.

Knowledge and understanding of the world

- Understanding cause and effect
- Using technology and switch work
- Forming positive relationships with adults and children
- Problem solving
- Working towards an end product.

Communication and language development

- Learning repetitive songs and rhymes
- Signing and using gestures
- Using clear, concise language
- Listening to and following instructions
- Encouraging children to vocalize and volunteer.

Physical development and movement

- Developing hand function skills (manipulation skills, using two hands together and individually)
- Developing whole body skills (e.g. crawling, jumping, stepping stones (stepping from mat to mat)).

Expressive and aesthetic development

- Singing, music and rhythm.

Emotional personal and social development

- Helping to create own snack or drink
- Dressing skills (socks and shoes on or off)
- Encouraging peer interaction
- Playing cooperatively, taking turns and sharing
- Building up self-confidence and self-esteem.

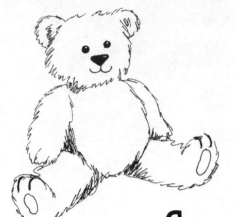

3

What is Sensory Processing?

What are our senses?

Before providing more detail about running the Fuzzy Buzzy Group programme, we will outline some more information about sensory processing and what it might look like in children who are experiencing sensory processing difficulties.

We all have seven senses that we use to gather information: sight, sound, smell, taste, touch, movement and body position.

Sight (visual sense)

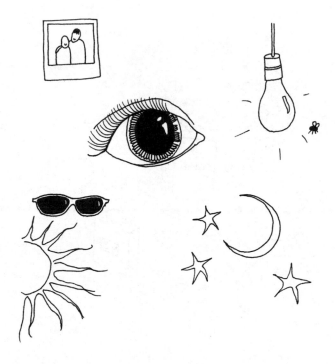

Sound (auditory sense)

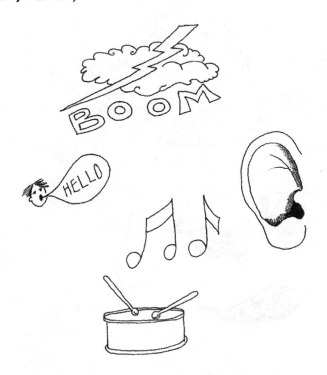

Smell (olfactory sense)

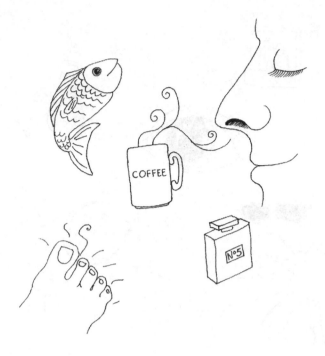

Taste (gustatory sense)

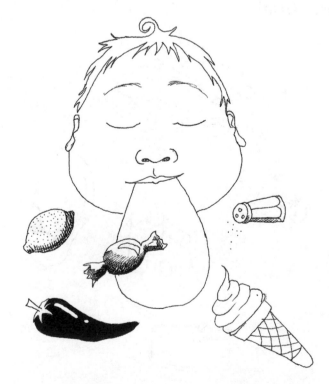

Touch (tactile sense)

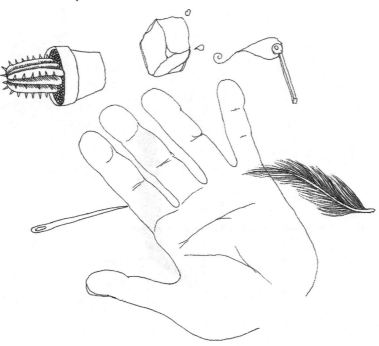

Movement (vestibular sense)

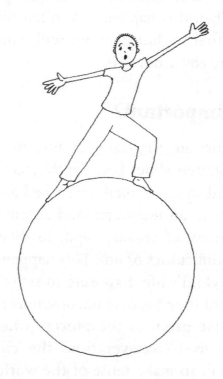

Body position (proprioception)

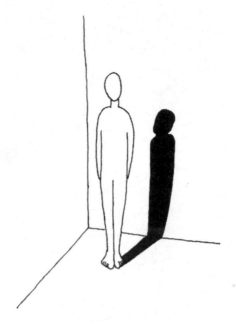

In order for us to carry out everyday actions, we take in information from our environment using all of our senses. These senses are processed in our brain and then interpreted. When this happens, we often react in an appropriate way, for example, if we touch a hot item, we will remove our hand, or if a noise is too loud, we may cover our ears.

Why are these senses important?

Our senses begin to function very early in life, in the womb. However, some senses may be forgotten about because they are 'unconscious senses' (think of how babies need to suck, smell, be rocked and cradled). All senses eventually work together in an integrated and automatic way. All children need to experience a variety of sensory input in their lives, whether they have sensory processing difficulties or not. This happens most importantly in the first eight years of a child's life. Exposure to sensory input and practice coordinate the senses until they become unconscious and forgotten.

Integration is the name given to the process whereby the brain gives meaning to the sensations it receives from the environment, responds accordingly and enables us to make sense of the world around us. Without this processing skill, the world can be a frightening and confusing place.

We all experience a great deal of environmental stimulation that either alerts us or calms us. For example, we might drink coffee to keep us awake, or we might listen to soft music to relax.

Sensory processing difficulties in children

Many children have problems with processing sensory information and may either seek out, or avoid, sensory experiences. However, children can improve their ability to process sensory information through engagement in appropriate activities and play. This helps to get the level of arousal 'just right'.

Symptoms often displayed by children with sensory integration difficulties, and which may be addressed through the use of a sensory programme, include the following:

- avoidance of touching certain textures, e.g. sticky items
- a need to touch or carry certain objects, e.g. blanket or soft toy
- sensitivity or abnormal response to light and sounds, e.g. covering eyes or ears
- high activity levels and a tendency to seek out movement, e.g. fidgeting or spinning
- poor concentration and attention to task
- delay in the development of self-care skills, e.g. dressing or feeding
- excessive eye flickering and grimacing
- poor behaviour and non-compliance.

These sensory processing experiences may involve the child being over-aroused or under-aroused:

Over-aroused (too much stimulation, child may withdraw from stimuli)

———————— The 'Just Right' arousal level ————————

Under-aroused (too little stimulation, child may seek out stimuli)

A reduction in the particular stimulation can help bring children *down* to their 'just right' level. An increase in the particular stimulation can help bring children *up* to their 'just right' level.

Children may also have difficulty maintaining a just right arousal level, which can lead to uncontrollable fluctuations from over- and under-sensory responses.

Listed below are examples of over-arousal and under-arousal sensory reactions which may be observed.

	Over-arousal	Under-arousal
Sight	Dislike of bright or flickering lights and visually busy environments	Attracted to light, fascinated with reflections, looks intently at objects or mirrors
Sound	Covers ears, light sleeper, dislikes sudden unexpected or loud noises	Bangs objects, seeks noisy environment, makes loud, rhythmic noises
Smell	Dislikes some smells, e.g. cleaning products, perfume	Smells objects, seeks strong odours, e.g. spicy, citrus
Taste	Fussy eater, uses tip of tongue for testing, gags or vomits easily, may prefer pureed foods	Eats anything, seeks strong flavours, mouths, licks non-food objects
Touch	Resists many textures, messy play, personal care, e.g. hair washing, certain clothes	Appears unaware of touch, low reaction to pain, unaware of messiness, e.g. runny nose
Movement	Dislikes being upside down or rough and tumble, intolerant of movement	Seeks out movement, e.g. spinning, rocking, jumping, flapping hands
Body position	Rough with toys, turns whole body to look at something, heavy pencil work	Low muscle tone, weak grip, lacks awareness of body positions

All seven senses identified are addressed within the programme and can be introduced within the sensory activities that form part of the structure of each session.

Encouraging appropriate responses

Therapeutic activities to facilitate child-centred treatment sessions should be carried out in a monitored and safe environment where children can be guided through activities which challenge their ability to respond appropriately to sensory input. Such activities help children experiencing processing difficulties to learn through routine and structure, thus enabling them to learn to organize their sensory systems and to make a successful, appropriate response.

If a child presents as avoiding sensory stimulus, treatment is likely to focus on *reducing* the sensitivity, or abnormal reaction, to sensory inputs such as sound or movement. If a child is showing behaviours which exhibit the need to seek certain sensations such as spinning or hand flapping, these inputs can be provided in a controlled and more 'socially acceptable' manner. It has been found that these strategies can help to decrease the behaviours in other situations.

Behaviour

When a child is upset by exposure to a certain noise or smell, an adult may become cross if the child refuses to comply with adult direction or displays what appears to be inappropriate behaviour. A vicious circle can then arise, as adult and child alike may become frustrated and tempers can flare.

What adults frequently do not understand is that the child is not necessarily intentionally behaving badly, but is actually finding it difficult to cope with a particular sensory experience. Therefore, it is important to be aware of the fact that the child may be displaying unwanted behaviours as a result of being unable to process, or correctly interpret, the sensory information being received. Behavioural difficulties and sensory difficulties often go hand-in-hand.

The purpose of this programme is to help practitioners and parents to understand and address what it is that the child finds difficult to process. It provides guidelines, strategies and activities to enhance coping mechanisms, while gently introducing the child to different sensory stimuli, in a happy and controlled manner.

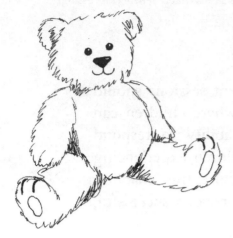

4

Child Development

It is helpful to have a good understanding of children's developmental stages when addressing sensory processing difficulties. As children grow and develop, they usually reach certain milestones and follow a similar sequence of developmental stages within an approximate time scale.

For anyone working with young children, it is important to recognize that children are unique individuals and they will develop at their own pace. The general guide below should not be used to determine what a specific child can or cannot do. It is not our intention to cause unnecessary anxiety when a child does not achieve a particular skill at a particular age.

Careful observation, liaising with parents and good communication with caregivers or other professionals are paramount when trying to determine the abilities of a child. Children may perform better on some days than others as many factors can affect their behaviour, such as anxiety, illness, lethargy. Numerous factors can delay development for a child, including a physical or learning impairment, or social factors such as abuse and/or neglect. However, understanding the typical pattern of child development will help you to determine whether a child is thriving or struggling in any given situation. This knowledge will help you to determine performance areas that a child may require further assistance with and may also help you work out how to promote their development in a skill area.

The developmental stages below are not definitive or extensive: only a handful of skills are listed for each area of development, in four different categories: cognitive, physical, play and sensory.

Children's developmental stages

By one year old, children may be able to do the following.

Cognitive	Look for a hidden toy, recognize familiar pictures, e.g. family members, understand 'No' and 'Bye bye', imitate adult noises, e.g. brrrr or a cough, babble loudly and continuously
Physical	Sit, crawl, bottom shuffle, stand holding onto furniture, use a pincer grasp, pass toys from one hand to the other, maintain hold of an object, e.g. rattle or piece of toast
Play	Make noises by banging objects, place toys into and out of boxes, play with stacking beakers and bricks, explore objects with their hands and mouth, enjoy rough and tumble, play alone
Sensory	Turn to the sound of their mother's voice or a sudden noise, mouth objects to explore them, use a comforter such as a blanket or dummy or pacifier, be very visually alert to their surroundings

By two years old, children may be able to do the following.

Cognitive	Point to body parts on request, imitate words that an adult says, understand basic instructions (e.g. kiss Mummy), use between 10 and 20 recognizable words, show interest in picture books
Physical	Walk confidently and without bumping into objects, squat to pick up toy from floor, climb up steps with one hand held, point at objects, build a tower with a few bricks, use a spoon, hold a pencil with a whole hand and scribble onto paper
Play	Play with posting boxes, shape sorters, screw and unscrew objects, sensory items, e.g. sand, dough and water, enjoy puppet and action games, begin to engage in imaginative play, e.g. putting dolly to bed, tolerate others playing beside them
Sensory	Recognize familiar people from a distance, recognize self in a mirror, enjoy being involved in messy play activities. Children tend not to take items to their mouth to explore any more

By three years old, children may be able to do the following.

Cognitive	Understand consequences, e.g. when they hurt someone else, speak over 200 words, form basic sentences, e.g. 'I want my teddy', know their full name, ask 'why' questions, say a few nursery rhymes, try to sing along to nursery rhymes
Physical	Walk up and down steps (one foot per step), propel trike with feet on floor, run confidently, climb outdoor apparatus, kick and throw a ball, jump two feet together from a step, turn single pages of a book, hold a pencil in a more refined grasp and copy lines and circles, build a tower of seven or more bricks
Play	Enjoy constructional play, e.g. building and transport toys, enjoy climbing, running, begin interacting with peers, further developed imaginative play, e.g. ironing clothes and hanging up, go shopping
Sensory	Recognize familiar people in photographs including themselves, point out minute details in picture books

By four years old, children may be able to do the following.

Cognitive	Match two or three primary colours, carry a simple conversation, count up to ten, remember and repeat nursery rhymes, master toilet training, show concern and empathy for others
Physical	Ride a trike using the pedals, throw and catch a ball, walk on tip toes, walk backwards and sideways, copy basic brick pattern, e.g. a bridge, draw a person's head and facial features, cut paper with scissors, eat using a fork
Play	Enjoy playing with jigsaw puzzles and trains, make models, turn take with peers as well as some time-alone playtime, join in imaginative play with other children, e.g. doctor and patient, enjoy craft activities, e.g. gluing/making a card, engage in games such as lotto and Kim's game (a test of observation and memory)
Sensory	Match and name two primary colours

By five years old, children may be able to do the following.

Cognitive	Count up to 20, often mix up fact with fiction, sort objects into categories, problem solve well, state first line of their address
Physical	Walk along a chalk line, bounce a ball, attempt climbing trees, run up and down steps (one foot per step), ride a tricycle with skill and turning handle bars with ease, thread very small beads onto a lace, hold a pencil in an adult manner, draw a person

| Play | Play elaborate role-play games, enjoy exercise, board games, floor games, arts and craft materials, draw objects and people, model dough or clay into objects, e.g. a snail |
| Sensory | Match and name four primary colours, maintain concentration to long detailed stories |

What is developmental delay?

Children with developmental delay may have a specific learning difficulty or a diagnosis such as Down syndrome. However, some children may not have an obvious disability but may have general difficulties learning tasks and remembering things. Many children have no specific diagnosis and there may be no clear explanation as to why the child is not functioning at the same level as his or her peer group.

There are many standardized tests that can be completed to determine whether a child is developmentally delayed (e.g. Movement ABC-2, Schedule of Growing Skills, Guide to Early Movement Skills, Griffiths Developmental Scale). Often, this is an inconsistent profile (by this we mean that a child may score well in some areas but not in others).

As children grow and develop, they need to be exposed to a range of different experiences. What they see, hear and play with is all vital in their development. Children with developmental delay may require more frequent and intense input or intervention than other children of a similar age, or they may have missed experiential opportunities, perhaps due to family circumstances. It is not too late to offer children an experience when they get a little bit older. A child with developmental delay often requires repetition and routine in order to learn new developmental skills. We believe that this programme provides such an opportunity.

Children learn by seeing and doing, which is why they benefit greatly from interacting in a fun activity with their peers. However, many children with developmental delay are isolated in their play and they may need support to enable them to interact with others. Some children with developmental delay may initially prefer to be a casual observer, but is important that they become active participants as soon as possible. Adult assistance can facilitate this process to ensure that the children can freely experience the activities on offer. A key strategy is to make the activity motivational. If children enjoy what is happening, they will want to do it again and again.

Adults can offer activities that will enhance children's play and ensure the activity is tailored to their specific needs. Not only can we offer support to a child and ensure activities are gauged at an appropriate level, but also we can offer praise and encouragement which, in turn, should develop a child's confidence and self-worth as well as the ability to carry out daily activities. As soon as there are suspicions that children may be behind in their developmental milestones, it is imperative that they are offered multiple opportunities to promote their sense of self-worth and self-confidence. It is important that children experience activities that they may have missed in order to help them reach their full potential. This should encompass play, posture, exposure to the senses, fine motor and oral motor skills. The skills offered in this programme are suitable for children from around two years of age as this is the age they are starting to play interactively and be more aware of other children.

As children with developmental delay may not be able to tell you verbally how they are feeling, keen observation is essential. Look closely at a child's facial expressions and reactions to give you an idea of how to respond.

If you feel comfortable doing it, it can be helpful to accompany words with signs and gestures, using not only facial expression, but also hands. Remember how gestures help if you are in a foreign country and do not speak a word of the language. The same goes for children who are struggling to understand what you are asking or saying. Gesture reinforces the verbal word and visual cues so the child has a better chance of following what is being asked or said.

Developmental age versus developmental stage

The group is designed to be suitable for children with developmental delay, and so it is more appropriate to look at what stage a child is functioning at rather than the actual age of the child. For example, a child may be seven years old but is presenting at the approximate age of a four-year-old. The programme would be appropriate and, most likely, very enjoyable for this child.

Children often go though certain types of age-related behaviour such as temper tantrums, often known as the 'terrible twos', where the child begins to become defiant and strong-willed around the age of two. However, if the child has a developmental delay, age-related behaviours are more likely to occur when the child is older, therefore not making them age-related!

Children who have a delay in their development will usually reach the

34   Copyright © Fiona Brownlee and Lindsay Munro 2010

typical development milestones expected of them, just at a considerably slower rate.

Developmental delay and typical characteristics

Children who are delayed may have a number of additional traits that can affect their learning. For example, they may

- have a short attention span
- be afraid to try new things
- be easily distracted
- prefer to play with younger children
- have difficulty working out new tasks or problem solving
- have difficulty retaining information
- play with toys or games often associated with younger children.

Physical or learning disabilities

A child who has a physical or cognitive disability may also not necessarily follow the typical developmental milestones. A child may meet some developmental stages on target but not others. Some children may achieve milestones later and some may never attain certain developmental milestones at all. This should be taken into consideration when determining the developmental stage that a child has reached.

Children with additional difficulties may need extra support and time in order to complete certain activities or learn new skills. Other factors may affect the development of a child with a physical or cognitive difficulty, such as the learning opportunities they are exposed to or offered. Children with impairments have the same basic needs as 'typically' developing children, but a child with a disability can often miss out essential opportunities and experiences. This can have a negative effect on the child forming relationships with others, learning new skills and engaging in physical, developmental and sensory activities.

If you are concerned about a child's development, for example if a child is not reaching normative stages, these concerns should be shared with the parent or carer.

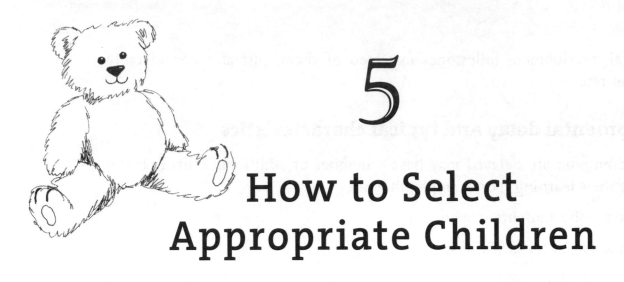

5
How to Select Appropriate Children

In order to assess whether a child may be suitable to participate in the group, the following inclusion and exclusion criteria may be used. Trust your instincts and be your own sensory detective. Behaviours that suggest a child will benefit from a Fuzzy Group are listed on pp.38–9.

Ideally, there should be no more than eight children in a Fuzzy Buzzy Group and, preferably, an adult allocated to each child (parental input would be helpful in this instance). Groups with more than eight children would make it too long for individual children to wait their turn.

The information in this chapter should help you to choose which children are appropriate to include in the group, but you will need to think about how to approach the parents for consent sensitively and appropriately. Where children and their parents are already known to you and it is acknowledged that they have sensory processing difficulties, it should be relatively straightforward. If the difficulty is not already recognized, then you will need to broach the idea with a lot of tact and diplomacy. In all cases, you should fully explain the purpose of the group to parents and how it may benefit their child.

Children diagnosed with sensory processing difficulties

Sensory processing difficulties can present in children who have, for example, been diagnosed as having a specific additional support need, such as developmental delay, cerebral palsy, attention deficit hyperactivity disorder, Down syndrome, neonatal abstinence syndrome, foetal alcohol syndrome or autism. The number of children being diagnosed with autism is increasing. Initially, they may exhibit the 'triad of impairments', that is poor communication, social skills and imagination. There is also a high correlation between autism and sensory processing difficulties; we believe that sensory processing difficulties should be included as the fourth impairment.

The earlier that intervention starts, the better for the developing brain. The brain is very flexible in the early years and neural pathways can be laid down, resulting in behavioural and motor patterns being created.

Children with additional support needs or who have disabilities often miss out on inclusive activities and later in life can become bored and lonely. If there are physical difficulties in a child, there is a higher chance that the normal sensory, rough-and-tumble times have been overlooked or omitted. Normal exploratory opportunities can be limited and consequently sensory input reduced. This can, although not always, mean that the children have poor sensory regulation.

In promoting friendship and offering opportunities to join in activities with others who may or may not have disabilities, the Fuzzy Buzzy Group provides these children with opportunities they may not normally have and helps them learn and have fun through repetition and exposure to the senses.

We are often asked if children with visual impairment would benefit from this group. The answer is a definite 'Yes'. Fuzzy Buzzy Groups are ideally suited for children who have limited vision. The contrasting textures, the songs, the familiar routine, all help children to understand their world, although they may need a little more encouragement and guidance than others in the group.

Premature babies, low birth weight babies, and those who have had a lot of hospitalization in their early years, may have had limited and infrequent contact with a familiar adult and may well be tactile defensive. They may also find textures unappealing or be reluctant to explore activities. These children will find the Fuzzy Buzzy Group beneficial.

Many children are intolerant of processing sensory information for no apparent reason and have no diagnosis. These include children who have been under-stimulated in their early years or have general global delay. Some behaviours may have also been learned from experience, for example if a child has been constantly told that something is 'dirty' or if a member of the family has exhibited sensory difficulties or inappropriate reactions and the child has witnessed this. There are many children who remain undiagnosed but who struggle to make sense of the world around them.

Behaviours that suggest a child will benefit from a Fuzzy Buzzy Group

Children may attend a sensory group if they present more than one of the following:

- Dislike touching everyday items set up for play in nursery or school, for example craft work, sand, slime, paint, dough, soil.

- Are sensitive to or display abnormal responses to sounds, such as a lawnmower, hairdryer, vacuum cleaner, screaming, bell ringing, music (tape, instrument or voice).

- Dislike being messy, such as having food traces on face or hands.

- Are very picky about the kinds of food they will eat.

- Are intrigued with lights or light switches.

- Constantly watch themselves in the mirror.

- Are fixated with spinning wheels or lining toys up.

- Are evasive with eye contact.

- Smell and mouth objects (beyond the developmental age for doing this).

- Are either too clingy or reject physical comfort or contact.

- Are sensitive or display abnormal responses to rough-and-tumble or outside play or gym.

- Become upset on car or bus journeys.

- Exhibit facial grimace when exposed to sensory stimuli.

- Present autonomic nervous system distress, for example face flushes, breathing rate increases when presented with a sense they dislike.

- Have problems coping with change of routine.

- Do not cope with new situations.

- Exhibit movements and coordination out of line with intellectual abilities.

- Display disruptive behaviours such as attention seeking, destruction.

- Have difficulty making friends.

- Are slow to follow and understand instructions.

- Are slow to speak.

- Have poor social interaction.

- Fail to understand or pick up unspoken clues from others.

Children unsuitable to attend a Fuzzy Buzzy Group

Children who may not be suitable for attendance at the group might include those who

- Have a very limited IQ level and may not be able to understand or carry out simple instructions, even with adult assistance.

- Are too young to be expected to comply with group activities (e.g. children younger than 18 months of age).

- Are at a developmental age at which it might be considered appropriate for the child to be sensory seeking. As a rough guide, it is normal for children to mouth and taste toys from around nine months. This behaviour gradually ceases by around two years of age.

Every child is an individual and should be taken on his or her own merit. When considering whether a child should attend the group, it is important to look at the whole child in order to determine suitability, for example do the child's sensory difficulties create a barrier to learning?

Involving parents

Partnership with parents is crucial. Always ask permission from the parents or carers before involving a child in the group (a consent form is provided in the Handouts section). It is important to explain to parents why you would like to involve their child in the programme and explain what benefits their child will receive from attending.

Parents' in-depth knowledge of their children is very important and useful. They may observe behaviours at home that are not always seen at the child's placement setting, which may help to provide a better understanding of the child's difficulties with sensory processing.

The ideal ratio is one adult to one child. Parents are often willing to participate, which can help them understand their child's difficulties and abilities and also give them ideas about how they can support their child at home.

The contact between parents whose children have similar issues also provides much needed peer support, even if it is in an informal manner. This should not be overlooked, as parents often report that they have a constant battle to find out about different agencies or what services are available. Informal chat between parents has been found to be extremely helpful.

6
Running the Group

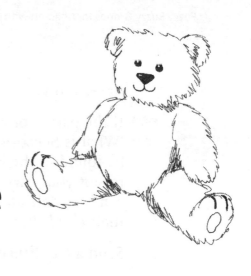

Preparing to run the group

Before you can run the group, you will need to carry out some planning – thinking about who will attend, what you want to do each week and when and where the sessions will take place. You will also need to speak to the parents of the children participating.

The group should run for no longer than one hour and fifteen minutes but timings can be adjusted according to your needs. The maximum number for the group is eight and the minimum number is three.

The routine, layout of the room and format of the group should remain the same for each session in order to allow the children to feel secure and to create continuity.

The illustration on p.43 is an example of how you could set out a room to run a Fuzzy Buzzy Group, familiarize yourself with the layout and also the guide to the seven different steps on pp.46–52 to develop a clear idea of what each session will involve. Think of an appropriate venue where you could run the group.

1. Identify the children who may be suitable for inclusion in the group (refer back to Chapter 5). Decide whether you want parents to attend or not.

2. Identify a lead person to run the group.

3. Talk with parents and carers to determine whether they would be happy for their child to participate in the group (and, if appropriate, whether the parent would like to come along with their child to help).

4. Having given thought to when and where to run the group, set the dates, times and venue, which need to be agreeable to all those participating.

5. If the parent or carer is in agreement, send out the Consent Form and the 'What is Sensory Processing?' handout (all forms, handouts and letter can be found in the Handout section). You may want to adapt the Consent Form to suit your own needs (approaching parents about their children attending can be a delicate matter). If the parent or carer chooses not to participate, their child should not be considered for the group.

6. Send a Confirmation Letter to each parent and carer.

7. Decide which sensory areas are to be addressed each week (consult the section 'Selecting sensory themes' on p.44) and choose the food to be provided at snack time. Record your plans on the Fuzzy Buzzy Session Planner, creating one for each of the eight sessions. Remember, these can be revisited if you find that you want to make changes to fit with the children's particular needs. Take care not to feature foods or materials to which any of the participating children are allergic.

8. At the end of the final session complete an Evaluation Form for every child in order to identify any improvements in the child's functional abilities. This will help to provide evidence of what you have covered and also any progress by the participating children.

Laying out the room for a Fuzzy Buzzy Group

The illustration overleaf shows how a room can be set up for Fuzzy Buzzy Group sessions. We found this particular layout most useful as it allows children to follow a regular routine: for Step 1 Hello, the children enter through the door and choose a mat on which to sit. Adults can sit on the floor beside the children to create one circle.

The children remain seated in the circle while exploring the sensory bags (Step 2 Sensory bags), using the liquidizer (Step 3 Drink preparation) and watching the teddies being placed into a pram or buggy and going away to hide (Step 4 Teddies go to hide). When the children have removed their socks and shoes, they make their way through a tunnel (optional) and travel along the sensory path to find their teddies (Step 5 Sensory path), then they have a picnic (Step 6 Snack time) before they go home (Step 7 Goodbye). The snack table could be set up with plates, cups, cutlery and food prior to the group starting.

The room does not need to be set up precisely as the illustration shows, but the following points are important:

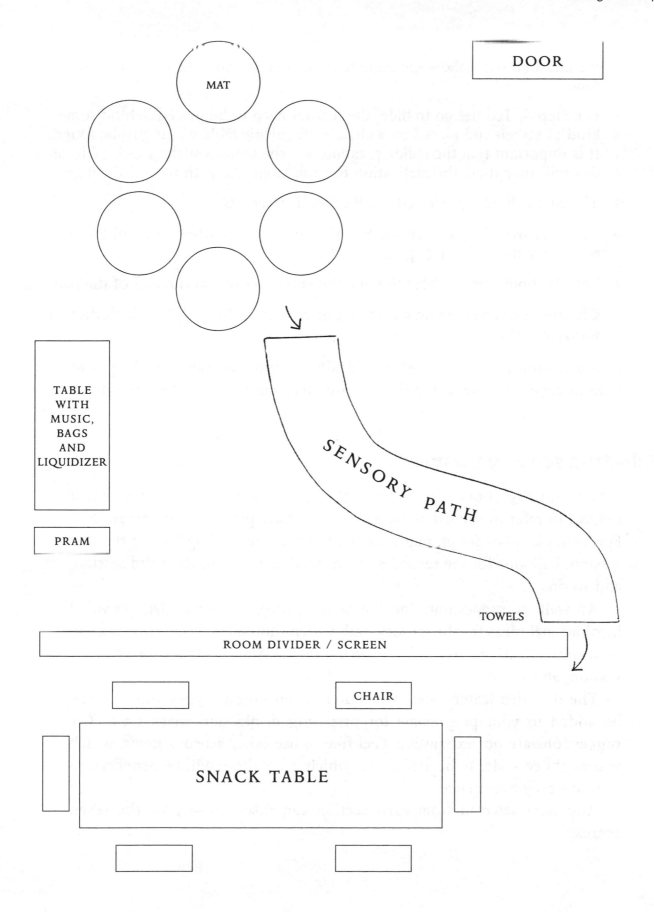

MAT

DOOR

TABLE
WITH
MUSIC,
BAGS
AND
LIQUIDIZER

PRAM

SENSORY PATH

TOWELS

ROOM DIVIDER / SCREEN

CHAIR

SNACK TABLE

- The room should be set up in exactly the same way for every session, so that the children will follow the same route and be in the same environment every time.

- For Step 4, Teddies go to hide, the teddies need to be placed behind some kind of screen and placed on a chair at the picnic table waiting to be found. It is important that the children cannot see the teddies at the snack table, as this will give them the motivation to walk along the path to find them.

- The room should be cleared of all other distractions.

- Be aware that the path can become slippery and wet when some of the sensory items are on it (e.g. foam and gel).

- Towels should be available to wipe the children's feet at the end of the path.

- Children can change into a spare set of clothes at the end if their clothes are messy or wet.

If you choose to use a tunnel it is ideally around two metres in length to help to create a sense of travelling a distance, and can be either straight or curvy.

Selecting sensory themes

When thinking about what sensory themes to introduce, you may find it helpful to refer to the list of suggestions we have provided (see pp.56–61). For example, play dough might be used in the sensory bag list for the first session, balloons for the second session, survival wrap for the third session, and so on.

As well as suggestions for the sensory bag, we have also provided inspirational ideas for the sensory path which should be varied from session to session – perhaps using foam for the first session, feathers for the next session, and so on.

The lists also feature some sweet and savoury food suggestions that can be added to your programme for preparing drinks and snack time. The suggestions are not exhaustive. Feel free to use other sensory items, which you might consider to be useful, and which you believe will be beneficial to a child's play experience.

Any item selected from each section can relate to any of the seven senses:

- sight
- sound
- smell
- taste
- touch
- movement
- body position.

For example, in one session, you may use play dough for the tactile sense (touch), choose the stepping stones for balance and movement, and use mint in the liquidizer for taste and smell.

Try to assess which sensory experiences the child will tolerate with ease and which sensory items the child will not tolerate easily, as you may wish to consider grading the sensory items that are introduced over each session.

For example, if a child has a dislike of messy play items but does not mind vibrations, you may choose to have a buzzy or pull string toy in the sensory bag on the first week rather than slime. It is hoped that over the eight sessions, when the child can predict what is about to happen through repetition and preparation, the child's anxieties will diminish and he or she will be more able to tolerate the sensory experience.

Final preparations before you run the session

Having organized when, where and how you will run your session, and thought about sensory activities, make sure you run through the following checklist:

- A person has been chosen to lead the session.

- It has been agreed which senses are to be introduced for the session and the reasons for including these in the programme.

- The room is set up prior to the children arriving.

- If required, the words of the songs are photocopied and displayed on the walls (see Handouts section).

- Parents and carers have received a copy of the plan for the day (and any future sessions), even if they are not attending in person.

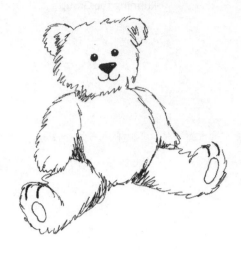

7

Now You Can Begin

What follows is a seven-step breakdown of the activities that you will do every time you run one of the eight Fuzzy Buzzy sessions.

Step 1 Hello

Aims of this step

- To signify the beginning of the group through song.

- To help the children focus on what is about to happen.

- To create group unity, e.g. by holding hands.

How to do it

1. Have the 'Fuzzy Buzzy Song' playing prior to the children entering the room (CD song 1) (see Handouts section for all songs). Place the song on 'repeat' and switch off the music only when all the children are sitting down on their mats. If your CD player does not have a repeat button, you could continue to sing the song when it has ended.

2. When everyone is seated in a circle, stop the music or singing.

3. Play and sing the song 'All Together Now' (CD song 2) while holding hands. Do not insist that the children hold hands if they are reluctant to do so but use gentle encouragement.

4. Stop the CD when the song has ended.

Useful notes

The children's familiarity with the 'Fuzzy Buzzy Song' is central to this step, and will develop with repeated sessions. The familiar song is comforting for the children as it signifies that they are going to have fun and that the group is about to begin. It is not important where in the circle each child chooses to sit, although the children may often choose to sit in the same place every week.

Step 2 Sensory bags

Aims of this step

- To promote anticipation: the song that starts off the activity acts as a signifier for the sensory activity about to be carried out.

- To introduce a new sensory activity in a fun manner.

- To promote joint awareness and participation by exploring the sense with the adult and other children.

- To develop fine motor skills such as pinch grip, using two hands together.

How to do it

1. The lead person hands out a sensory bag to each child. Each sensory bag contains a different item, but all of the items should be an example of the same sense (e.g. squishy, crackly). These should be passed around the circle to each adult accompanying a child.

2. Play and sing the song 'Let Us Have a Look' (CD song 3) and begin to explore the contents of the bag. Do not force any child to touch the item.

3. Praise any exploration of the item and make it fun. The adult should explore the item with the child in a calm, interested fashion.

4. When it is time to put the bags away (after approximately ten minutes) encourage the child to help put the item back into the bag. Say, 'Put it away' when instructed by the lead person.

5. Pass the sensory bags back to the lead person and remove from sight.

Useful notes

For the purpose of the group we purchased silver plastic bubble pack bags from a local stationer and placed the sensory item within it. The bag you use does not need to be this particular type. Use whatever you can find, provided it is not transparent.

In advance of the group starting, the sensory item for the session should have been chosen and placed in the bag. It is essential to know the properties of the object being presented, for example balloons can make squeaky noises and fly away or be blown up and deflated. Experiment before beginning.

It is important to observe the children's response and decide on the length of time to play with the item. For example, if the children are becoming bored with the item, it might be time to put it away or exchange it with someone else's in the group. If the child displays an adverse reaction to the stimuli, be prepared to persevere and try to present the item in different ways, even it means the adult playing with the item and the child just watching.

Step 3 Drink preparation

Aims of this step

- To build up tolerance to the sound of a liquidizer or blender.

- To introduce different tastes and smells in a fun manner.

- To build up sequencing in a task; pour in liquid, add flavour or fruit, put lid on, press button, pass on to next child.

- To promote turn-taking and peer awareness.

- To develop listening skills.

How to do it

1. Having previously selected a taste for the session, let each child have the opportunity to smell, touch and taste the ingredients prior to placing them into the liquidizer jug. The adult should also smell and taste the food.

2. Warn each child that there is going to be a big noise and say 'Ready, Steady, Go!' before the switch is activated, in order to build up anticipation. When you have demonstrated what happens, offer each child an opportunity to press the switch.

3. Praise any effort made. Everyone should clap and say, 'Well done ———' for each attempt.

4. If a child refuses to participate, calmly pass the switch to the next child.

5. When everyone has had a turn, ask if anyone wants to press the switch again.

6. When all the children who want to participate have had their turn, say 'Finished'.

7. Remove the liquidizer and tell the children that they can taste the drink at snack time.

Useful notes

Use a blender to make the snack drink for the day. An adult should be responsible for controlling the liquidizer and assisting the child to press the button (take care with electrical leads). Prior to starting, have the basic liquid already in the liquidizer or jug. All that needs to be added is the taste or ingredient for that session, for example banana, chocolate powder (we have provided some suggestions on p.63–64).

Do not leave the choice of the drink to the last minute and be aware that the children may be apprehensive about tasting, smelling or adding the ingredient to the liquidizer. Some children dislike the noise of the liquidizer and may be reluctant to press the switch. If this happens, the adult can do it for them and prepare them for what is expected. It is hoped that the child will learn to tolerate the noise of the liquidizer over the course of the different sessions. However, a whisk or spoon could be used as an alternative to mix the ingredients of the drink together if the noise is too unbearable for some children.

Step 4 Teddies go to hide

Aims of this step

- To promote an understanding of 'object permanence', that is, understanding that when a toy disappears, it has not gone for good.

- To help develop memory, visual scanning and recognition. The children have to find their own teddy sitting at the table after they have crawled through the tunnel and walked along the sensory path.

How to do it

1. Play the 'Fuzzy Buzzy Song' as background music (CD song 1).

2. The lead person should explain that all the teddies are going to hide and the children should say or wave 'Bye bye'. The teddies are placed in a pram, wheeled away and put on the chairs around the picnic table. The teddies should not be visible to the children.

Useful notes

This can be a distressing activity for a child, especially if it is their own teddy rather than one belonging to the nursery or provided for the session. Children can be reluctant to part from their teddy, especially during the first few sessions of the programme. Do not force this: if they refuse to be separated, tell them they can take their teddy with them on the journey down the sensory path later on.

Step 5 Sensory path

Aims of this step

- To develop anticipation, e.g. removal of socks and shoes.

- To develop dressing skills by assisting removal of shoes and socks.

- To develop body and spatial awareness by crawling through a tunnel.

- To experience a variety of different senses through the children's legs and feet.

How to do it

1. The lead person should explain that everyone has to go and find their teddies. Play and sing the song 'Socks and Shoes' (CD song 4).

2. All children should remove their socks and shoes (or be assisted to remove them). Adults may wish to join in with the activity, as this can be reassuring for apprehensive children.

3. Encourage the children (and adults if possible) to crawl through the tunnel (information on how to source material for a tunnel is given on pp.59–60). If some children resist, try placing the tunnel over the children's heads while they are standing.

4. Everyone should walk along the path, one by one. Initially, the lead person should demonstrate what to do. Praise each child for any efforts made, even if they are minimal. This may be adapted with regard to the individual child's abilities, for example the child can crawl if unable to walk or the child may wish to have both hands held.

5. An adult should be positioned at the other end of the path to encourage the child along.

6. An adult should use a towel to wipe the excess mess, e.g. foam, off the children's feet at the end of the path.

7. When everyone has attempted this activity, they are then allowed behind the screen to find their teddies and sit down for their picnic (the children's socks and shoes are still off at this point).

Useful notes

Depending on the children's cognitive level, the sense that is put on the path could be called 'snow' (for foam) or 'water' (for gel), rather than just 'foam' or 'jelly' or 'bubble pack'. This can add to the sense of fun and play. Some children will want to walk along the path again, which is fine. However, they should be reminded to wait and let other children take their turn first. Sometimes it is not the texture that the child dislikes but the fact that it is slippery and cold. The children may feel insecure and unsafe. Lend a reassuring hand if necessary and be careful that the children do not fall.

Step 6 Snack time

Aims of this step

- To broaden their experience of taste, texture and consistency of food and drink.

- To build up sitting tolerance.

- To develop self-care skills in eating and drinking, e.g. scooping and cutting.

- To develop peer awareness and interaction.

- To introduce basic table manners through example.

How to do it

1. Gently encourage the children to taste the food and drink.

2. Leave the food and drink on the main table for the children to explore at their own pace.

3. Encourage children to remain seated for the duration of snack time, if possible.

4. Adults should fill in a Feeding Checklist (see Handouts section) for each child.

5. Adults should complete a Sensory/Behaviour Form (see Handouts section) for each child.

6. After the 'picnic', the children should put on their socks and shoes and return to their mats. (The path has already been removed or screened off.)

Useful notes

Feeding checklists and sensory/behaviour forms are useful for keeping a record of what children have explored and their reactions to different sensory experiences. They can be useful to refer to when choosing sensory experiences for future sessions.

Step 7 Goodbye

Aims of this step

- To develop recognition of the end of the group through the familiar song.

- To praise and offer a reward for attending and participating in the group.

How to do it

1. Play and sing the song 'Goodbye' (CD song 5).

2. Give a handmade teddy bear badge or sticker to each child (see Handouts section for templates that can be used) and praise.

Useful notes

The children may be tired by this point, especially in the initial sessions when the activities are new and unfamiliar. This is the time to relax and spend some time praising the children. Also remind the children that they will be returning to play again in the Fuzzy Buzzy Group. All children should receive a teddy bear badge or sticker, regardless of how much they have participated.

Once all seven steps have been completed, the session has finished. At the end of the final session, the Evaluation Form Sheet should be completed to assess the child's performance and to determine whether the child has made any improvements. Take particular care to note whether the parents now have an improved understanding of why their child behaves as he or she does. If they do not, ensure that they are provided with support to improve their knowledge – perhaps by putting them in touch with a local occupational therapist.

General tips for the session leader

- Always make it fun!

- If any children resist any sensory activities, respect their wishes.

- Try to run the group in a way that turns the activities into a game.

- Singing can be used by adults as a distraction from sensory activities if a child is uncomfortable.

- Schedule activities in such a way that periods of sitting are alternated with periods of movement.

- Be flexible! You can incorporate motivational toys into the play so that the child is engaged and wants to participate.

- Speak to all participating adults beforehand to make sure they understand what they will be doing and what behaviour works most effectively (see 'General tips for adults involved in running a session' in the next section. It is also available in a photocopiable form in the Handouts section).

General tips for adults involved in running a session

Adults who are involved in the group should work together to plan, deliver and evaluate the activities. They should endeavour to:

- Keep the children calm but interested in the activities. Children may be more susceptible to becoming distressed or excitable when attending the group.

- Monitor the children closely during each group session and evaluate each child's performance weekly, adapting further sessions accordingly. Children may display signs of being overwhelmed by the environment.

- Show no adverse reactions to the textures being introduced. The aim is to make the children feel at ease and demonstrate that it can be fun to play with the textures presented.

- Encourage and support the children to join in but do not force them to touch any items if they are unhappy to do so. The adult should touch the item instead and calmly show interest. Try to reintroduce the item tactfully at a later time.

- Talk to the children reassuringly and let them know what is about to happen.

- Speak in a soothing, gentle manner.

- If you are able to, use signs or simple gestures to help the children focus on what is being said. If you do use signs, ensure that they are used consistently by all adults in all sessions to avoid the children getting confused.

- Give the children time to approach activities in their own time. Do not rush them.

- For the sensory bag activity and any other appropriate times, encourage the children to touch the item and then to put it away. This allows the children to feel in control.

- Walk with the children along the path, hand in hand, in the gross motor 'sensory path' section.

- Always praise any effort made; you can even offer praise at times when the child is not doing anything troublesome, e.g. 'Good sitting!', 'That's nice playing!'

- Finally, make sure you have fun, enjoy the group and build up relationships!

Watching out for over-stimulation

Children may become over-stimulated when engaged in sensory activities. The warning signs can be subtle and may be displayed by a child

- grimacing

- trying to escape

- vocalizing in protest

- becoming frozen or rigid

- generally being upset or crying

- displaying excessive eye flickering or yawning.

Look out for these signs and, if you see them, try to calm and reassure the child.

8
Finding
Sensory Materials

Start building a sensory bank before you begin the group. You will find that a lot of sensory materials can be found at very low cost. If you mention you are running a sensory group to colleagues and friends, you are likely to find you are inundated with useful sensory things; it is surprising how word spreads.

What may be junk to some people may be treasure to you. It is worthwhile asking local shopkeepers if they could give you any unwanted stock. Factories are often willing to donate goods that may be surplus to their requirements but helpful for the group. We obtained new carpet samples from a local shop for the children to sit on at the start of the programme.

We have deliberately tried to obtain all sensory items from general toyshops, stationers, pharmacies and so on rather than from specialized toy retailers, which tend to be more expensive. However, a list of specialist suppliers in the UK, United States and Australia is provided later (see pp.66–68).

Objects useful for sensory activities can be found in museum shops, joke shops, garden centres, craft shops, home improvement stores, and around the classroom or home. It is amazing what can be found, especially at particular times of year such as Halloween or Christmas. It is not necessary to stick rigidly to the items suggested as these can be substituted with your own ideas. Resourcefulness and imaginative adaptation of everyday objects can usefully supplement resources specifically purchased for the activities.

Listed below are suggestions for themed activities for different sessions. Photocopy the Fuzzy Buzzy Session Planner (see Handouts section), fill in the blanks to suit your needs and begin. If you can think of additional sensory activities, add them to the list.

Many of the suggestions listed below can be used in both the fine and gross motor activities. While the material for activities is designed to be used as part of a structured programme, you may also find it useful as a 'dip in' resource for one-off activity ideas and inspiration.

The order in which you introduce different sensory activities does not matter: touch can be followed by sound, then vibration. If the group of children all have particular issues with sound it may be sensible to just concentrate on introducing sound activities only and omitting some of the other senses.

Resources list: the sensory bags

Activity	Sense	Where to purchase
Bubble pack bags (to contain items)	Visual/auditory	Post office, stationers
Sealable bags to contain items	Visual	Supermarket
Double-sided sticky tape	Tactile	Stationers
Bubble wrap	Auditory	Stationers/protective packaging
Shredded paper	Auditory/Visual	Offices
Wadding	Tactile	Sewing shops/quilters
Hair gel (put inside a sealable bag)	Tactile	Pharmacy
Elastic bands	Tactile	Stationers
Chalk	Tactile/Visual	Stationers
Foam discs	Tactile/Visual	Stationers
Stickyback plastic	Tactile/Visual	Stationers
Cling film	Tactile	Supermarket
Sticky spider light	Visual/Tactile	Supermarket
Balloons (safe use essential)	Visual/Auditory	Toy shop
Rubber-faced finger puppets (and spoon)	Visual/Tactile	Toy shop

Activity	Sense	Where to purchase
Slime (see p.61)	Tactile	DIY
Ooze	Tactile	Toy/joke shops
Gluck (pretend jelly) or pretend mud (see p.61)	Tactile	DIY/toy/joke shops
Scented gluck (see p.61)	Olfactory/Tactile	DIY
Hair gel	Olfactory/Tactile	Supermarket, pharmacy
Shaving foam (pretend cream)	Olfactory/Tactile	Supermarket
Pull string or vibrating toys	Visual/Tactile	Toy/pet shops
Noisy putty	Auditory/Tactile	Toy shop
Rainbow or air putty	Tactile/Joint awareness	Specialist supplier
Face paints	Visual/Tactile	Toy shop
Jelly/Jello	Tactile/Visual/Gustatory	Supermarket
Mud or soil	Tactile	Garden
Glue	Tactile/Olfactory	Stationers, supermarket
Sticky tape	Tactile	Stationers
Paint	Tactile/Visual	Toy shop
Sensory balls (Koosh)	Tactile	Toy shop
Battery-operated fans	Tactile/Visual	Hardware shop, pharmacy
Battery-operated toothbrushes	Tactile/Visual	Pharmacy
Rainbow torches or coloured cellophane over a torch	Visual	Stationers
Rubber octopus (or similar 'toy') soap holder	Tactile/Auditory	Pharmacy
Silver ball chains	Tactile/Visual	Hardware shop, DIY store
Whoopee cushion	Auditory	Joke/toy shops

Activity	Sense	Where to purchase
Cardboard or plastic tubing	Auditory	A plumber may give you some, or wrapping paper or kitchen roll tube
Survival wrap (can be used in a parachute game)	Visual/Auditory	Camping store (or from an exhausted marathon runner!)
Empty spray bottles or watering can	Tactile	General stores
Plastic bottle half filled with water and sparkle	Visual/Auditory	Stationers
Fibre-optic torches	Visual	General stores, toy shops
Strips of Velcro (hook-and-loop fasteners and felt) (try to get it in different colours)	Tactile/Auditory	General stores, fabric shop
Silver inner lining from a wine box	Olfactory/Visual/Auditory	Supermarket or wine merchant (make sure all the wine is drunk first!)
Magnets: fishing games, fridge magnets	Visual	Stationers, cook shop
Lengths of plastic tubing with marbles or beads inside	Visual/Auditory	Pet shop (tubing for fish tanks)
Body massage cream	Tactile/Olfactory	Pharmacy
Sticky wall creepers	Tactile/Visual	Toy shop
Stress balls	Tactile	Toy shop, stationers
Foil strips (sheets of foil may need to be shredded)	Tactile/Visual	Stationers
Hair cream	Olfactory/Tactile	Pharmacy
Self-adhesive putty	Tactile	Stationers, supermarket
Bubble wrap	Tactile	Stationers
Dough (see p.61)	Tactile	DIY

Resources list: the tunnel and the sensory path

The items in parentheses are suggestions for imaginative play. The first couple in the list are specifically for the tunnel part of the sensory path.

Activity	Sense	Where to purchase
Tunnel	Visual/Joint awareness/Vestibular	General toy shops or specialist suppliers such as ROMPA (see p.67)
Cardboard boxes (for the tunnel)	Joint awareness	Old packaging
Black bin bags	Tactile/Auditory	Supermarket
Bubble pack	Tactile/Auditory	Post office, stationers, empty packaging
Corrugated cardboard	Tactile	Stationers
Cork tiles	Tactile	Carpet shop, department store
Sheepskin	Tactile	Carpet shop, department store
Sandpaper	Tactile	Homeware shop, DIY store
Rubber sheeting	Tactile	Medical supplier
Rolls of wallpaper	Tactile	Hardware shop, or DIY store
Sheets of foam with soap and water	Tactile	Foam centre
Paint with sand (washed, not builder's) spread on path	Tactile	Garden centre
Dried lentils or dried peas spread on path	Tactile	Supermarket
Cooked spaghetti with oil added (worms)	Tactile	Supermarket
Feathers	Tactile	If you don't happen to know of an obliging duck or hen, deconstruct an old feather pillow!

Activity	Sense	Where to purchase
Wobble boards (stepping stones)	Joint awareness/ Vestibular	Specialist supplier such as Homecraft (see p.66)
Survival sheet/ space blanket (thunder/wind)	Visual/Auditory	Camping shops, running shop, specialist supplier
Hairdryer (wind)	Auditory/Tactile	Electrical shop, pharmacy, department store
Talcum powder (frost)	Olfactory/Tactile	Pharmacy
Shaving foam (snow)	Olfactory/Tactile/ Visual	Pharmacy
Blue hair gel (water)	Olfactory/Tactile/ Visual	Supermarket, Pharmacy
Wet and dry sand (beach)	Tactile	Toy shop
Soft play equipment, e.g. roll, wedge	Vestibular Joint awareness	Specialist supplier such as ROMPA or TFH (see p.67–68)
Papier mâché (see recipe below)	Tactile	Supermarket

Sensory item recipes

To keep the sensory bags clean, you could place some of the items into a separate polythene lining, such as a sealable food bag. Messy materials may also be put straight on to the sensory path for the gross motor activity section.

Papier Mâché

Ingredients: newspapers, flour, water

1. Tear newspapers into shreds and dip into flour and water paste (see Gluck recipe).

2. Children can help if possible with tearing newspapers and mixing paste.

3. Experiment with quantities to achieve the desired texture. Aim to achieve a sloppy texture.

Gluck

Ingredients: two parts cornflour to one part water. Food colorings and scents may be added to the gluck.

Dough

Ingredients: 1 cup of flour, 2 teaspoons of cream of tartar, ¼ cup of salt, 1 tablespoon of vegetable oil, 1 cup of water. Food colouring and flavouring may be added (e.g. peppermint).

1. Put ingredients into a pan, stir and cook over heat for a few minutes.

2. Remove from heat and knead.

Jelly/Jello

Follow instructions on the packet.

Choose strong-scented, brightly coloured flavours, e.g. strawberry or orange.

Slime

Ingredients: 2 cups of soap flakes and ½ cup of water

1. Add soap flakes to water and mix until soap flakes have blended.

2. Measurements can be adjusted in order to achieve the right consistency.

9
Choosing Sensory Food and Drink

Use a range of different types of food and drink over the eight sessions, such as fruity, scented, soft, crunchy, sweet and savoury. Remember to note the children's reactions on the weekly Feeding Checklist (see Handouts section), for example enjoyment, aversion, gagging, asking for more.

Equipment for preparing the food and drink

We generally use a liquidizer in order to make the drink recipes. Appropriate switches and control units can be purchased from specialist suppliers (see p.66–68) including Don Johnston (www.donjohnston.com) or ROMPA (www.rompa.com). However, it may be suitable for some children to activate the liquidizer using the switch on the unit itself.

It is important to remember always to keep leads and power points away from the children, and consider using a safe extension lead.

Food suggestions

When thinking about food and drink to use, make sure you have checked all participating children's food allergies and avoid using foods containing any ingredients to which they are allergic. Remember that some food and drink containing a lot of sugar, caffeine or additives may cause hyperactivity.

Savoury	Sweet
Biscuits/cookies	Jam/jelly
Corn snacks	Jelly/jello
Oatcakes	Chocolate spread
Cheese crackers	Peanut butter
Bread sticks	Rice pudding
Butter	Custard
Dips, e.g. houmous, salsa	Yoghurt
Crisps/chips	Fruit
Cheese	Honey
Water biscuits	Syrup
Vegetable sticks	Apple sauce
Chutney	Pancakes
Wafer	Trifle
Cereal	Ice cream
Nuts	Ice poles/ice lollies
Prawn crackers	
Tortilla	
Marmite/vegemite	

Drink suggestions

Milk

Milkshakes and smoothies

Fizzy juice or water

Chocolate drinks

Coffee

Frozen drinks or yoghurts

Warm malt drink

Water (sparkling or still or tap)

Tea or iced tea

Cola floats (add ice cream to cola)

Ice cubes added to water or juice

Using the liquidizer

1. Put the liquid base (e.g. milk or yoghurt) into the liquidizer first.

2. Children can take it in turns to help to pour it into the liquidizer.

3. Each child adds some prepared fruit, ice, ice cream or individual sachet or spoonful of flavouring to the liquidizer.

4. Use your imagination as to what can be added to the base, for example fruits in season or even fruit grown or picked by the children.

10
Helpful Resources

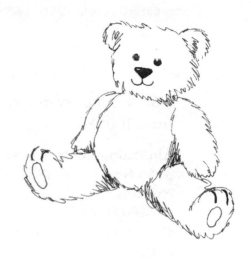

We have listed some useful books and suppliers worth investigating if you want to get some more ideas for sensory activities, or purchase particular sensory materials. We have tried to include suppliers from around the world, though many will deliver overseas.

Books

Blose, D.A. and Smith, L.L. (1995) *Thrifty Nifty Stuff for Little Kids*. Tucson, AZ: Communicaton Skill Builders.

Cooke, J. (2004) *Early Sensory Skills*. Bicester, UK: Speechmark.

Cribbon, V., Lynch, H., Bagshawe, B. and Chadwick, K. (2003) *Sensory Integration Information Booklet: A Resource for Parents and Therapists*. Greystones, Co., Wicklow, Ireland: Ross Print Services.

Dickinson, P. and Hannah, L. (1998) *It Can Get Better. A Guide for Parents and Carers*. London: National Autistic Society.

Hong, C.S., Gabriel, H. and St John, C. (2002) *Sensory Motor Activities for Early Development*. Bicester, UK: Speechmark.

Inamura, K.N. (1998) *Sensory Integration for Early Intervention: A Team Approach*. San Antonio, TX: Therapy Skill Builders.

Kranowitz, C.S. (2005) *The Out-of-Sync Child: Recognizing and Coping with Sensory Processing Disorder*. New York: Penguin.

Legge, B. (2002) *Can't Eat, Won't Eat: Dietary Difficulties and Autistic Spectrum Disorders*. London: Jessica Kingsley Publishers.

Warger, C.L. and Heflin, L.J. (1994) *Managing Behaviors: A Therapist's Guide*. Texas: AZ: Communication Skill Builders.

Wheeler, M. (2007) *Toilet Training for Individuals with Autism or Other Developmental Issues*. Arlington, TX: Future Horizons.

Specialist sensory suppliers

(All websites were accessed on 6 June 2009)

Abilitations Multisensory
3155 Northwoods Pkwy
Norcross,
GA 30071, USA
Customer service, toll free, tel: +1 800 850 8603
International fax: +1 770 263 0897
Evan Siegel: +1 800 444 5700 (ext. 7295)
Email: esiegel@sportime.com
www.abilitations.com
Provide information, solutions and equipment to improve the lives of special needs children.

Autism Teaching Tools
1107 East Allen
Tahlequah
OK 74464, USA
www.autismteachingtools.com
Practical source of information and teaching tips for working with special learners.

Baker Ross
2–3 Forest Works
Forest Road
Walthamstow
London E17 6JF, UK
www.bakerross.co.uk
Provide a catalogue of children's craft ideas and arts and crafts supplies.

Don Johnston
Tel (US and Canada): +1 800 999 4660
Tel (US and global): +1 847 740 0749
Email: info@donjohnston.com
www.donjohnston.com
Products and expertise for learners with reading and writing difficulties.

Early Years Education Resources
Gregory Street,
Hyde,
Cheshire SK14 4SG, UK
www.nesarnold.co.uk
Providers of school classroom equipment.

Homecraft
Nunn Brook Road
Huthwaite, Sutton in Ashfield
Nottinghamshire
NG17 2HU, UK
www.homecraft-roylan.com
Providers of rehabilitation products.

Indomed Pty Ltd
41 Forsyth St
O'Connor,
WA 6163, Australia
Tel: +61 (08) 9331 6711
Freecall: +61 1800 884 634
Fax: +61 (08) 9331 6722
Email: info@indomed.com.au
www.indomed.com.au
Free design and advice on equipment for setting up sensory rooms.

Kidscope Education
The Old Mill
Tricketts Lane
Willaston
Nantwich CW5 6PZ
Tel: +44 (0) 1270 567333
Fax: +44 (0) 1270 629295
Email: office@kidscopeeducation.co.uk
www.kidscopeeducation.co.uk
UK nationwide suppliers of arts and craft materials.

KidScope Toys
Email: contactus@kidscopetoys.com
www.kidscopetoys.com
Suppliers of educational and therapeutic toys.

Learning Development Aids
Pintail Close
Victoria Business Park
Nottingham NG4 2SG, UK
www.LDAlearning.com
Provide effective solutions to teaching and learning issues, from challenging behaviour to dyslexia.

Mike Ayres Design and Development Ltd
The Paddocks
Dore
Sheffield S17 3LD, UK
Tel: +44 (0) 114 235 6880
Fax: +44 (0) 114 235 6881
Email: enquiry@mike-ayres.co.uk
www.mike-ayres.co.uk
Design, provision and installation of soft play environments.

Mindstretchers
The Warehouse
Rossie Place
Auchterarder
Perthshire PH3 1AJ, UK
Tel: +44 (0) 1764 664409
Fax: +44 (0) 1764 664409
Email: enquiries@mindstretchers.co.uk
www.mindstretchers.co.u
Provide educational materials to help children learn in a multi-sensory and creative environment.

Perfectly Happy People
93 Bollo Lane
Chiswick London W4 5LU, UK
www.thebabycatalogue.com
Toys and useful products for parents and babies.

Promedics
Moorgate Street
Blackburn
Lancashire BB2 4PB, UK
www.promedics.co.uk
Providers of aids for daily living.

ROMPA®
Goyt Side Road
Chesterfield
Derbyshire S40 2PH, UK
Tel: +44 (0) 1246 211777
Fax: +44 (0) 1246 221802
www.rompa.com
Innovative catalogue of products designed for children with sensory impairments of all ages.

The Sensory Company International Ltd
Broad Lane Business Centre
Westfield Lane
South Elmsall WF9 2JX, UK
Tel: +44 (0) 845 838 2233
Fax: +44 (0) 845 838 2234
Email: webinfo@thesensorycompany.co.uk
www.thesensorycompany.co.uk
Design and manufacture 90 per cent of their sensory products for those who have learning difficulties.

Sensory Plus
(Part of Kirton Healthcare Group)
23 Rookwood Way
Haverhill
Suffolk CB9 8PB, UK
Freephone: +44 (0) 800 212709
Tel: +44 (0) 1440 705352
Fax: +44 (0)1440 706199
Email: enquiries@sensoryplus.co.uk
www.sensoryplus.co.uk
Large catalogue of sensory tools, equipment and environments.

SpaceKraft
Titus House
29 Saltaire Road
Shipley
West Yorkshire BD18 3HH, UK
Tel: +44 (0) 1274 581007
Fax: +44 (0) 1274 531966
www.spacekraft.co.uk
Suppliers of a range of sensory products for use in a sensory environment.

Special Direct
Park Lane Business Park
Kirkby-in-Ashfield
Nottinghamshire NG17 9GU
Tel: +1 (0) 800 318 686
Fax: +1 (0) 800 137 525
Email: sales@specialdirect.com
www.specialdirect.com
Well conceived products, specialising in
multi-sensory tools and multi-sensory
environments.

TFH Special Needs Toys
5–7 Severnside Business Park
Severn Road
Stourport-on-Severn
Worcestershire DY13 9HT, UK
Tel: +44 (0) 1299 827820
Fax: +44 (0) 1299 827035
www.tfhuk.com / www.specialneedstoys.
com/USA
Specialise in toys for children with
additional needs for learning.

Useful Handouts, Templates and Forms

All the following handouts, templates and forms may be photocopied for personal use when running a Fuzzy Buzzy Group.

Consent Form

Dear   Date:

From _____ we will be running a small group for children called the 'Fuzzy Buzzy Group'.

The purpose of this group is to help children who have sensory difficulties, developmental delay and/or behavioural issues to cope with carrying out everyday activities.

We have enclosed some information on sensory processing, which should help you understand why we think your child will benefit from attending such a group.

This group will run for ____ weeks at _____ from _____. There will be a snack time for the children and the emphasis is on fun and active participation.

By completing the form below and returning it no later than _____, your child will be put forward for selection to attend the group. You may also be invited to accompany your child.

You will be notified whether or not your child has been confirmed to attend the group by _____.

Yours sincerely,

Parent/carer's name: _____

Child's name: _____

Address:_____

_____

_____

_____

Telephone number:_____

Delete as applicable:

I agree for my child to participate in this group   Yes/No

The group involves children eating and drinking, and exploring different sensory materials. Please specify any dietary requirements and any allergies below:

_____

_____

_____

_____

_____

_____

Please return this form no later than _____

to _____

Signature: _____   Date: _____

Thank you

What is Sensory Processing?

What are our senses?

This handout is designed to provide you with some information about what sensory processing is and how children can experience sensory processing difficulties.

We all have seven senses that we use to gather information: sight, sound, smell, taste, touch, movement and body position.

Sight (visual sense)

Sound (auditory sense)

Smell (olfactory sense)

Taste (gustatory sense)

Touch (tactile sense)

Movement (vestibular sense)

Body position (proprioception)

In order for us to carry out everyday actions, we take in information from our environment using all of our senses. These senses are processed in our brain and then interpreted. When this happens, we often react in an appropriate way, for example, if we touch a hot item, we will remove our hand, or if a noise is too loud, we may cover our ears.

Why are these senses important?

Our senses begin to function very early in life, in the womb. However, some senses may be forgotten about because they are 'unconscious senses' (think of how babies need to suck, smell, be rocked and cradled). All senses eventually work together in an integrated and automatic way.

All children need to experience a variety of sensory input in their lives, whether they have sensory processing difficulties or not. This happens most importantly in the first eight years of a child's life. Exposure to sensory input and practice coordinate the senses until they become unconscious and forgotten.

We all experience a great deal of environmental stimulation that either alerts us or calms us. For example, we might drink coffee to keep us awake, or we might listen to soft music to relax.

Sensory processing difficulties in children

Many children have problems with processing sensory information and may either seek out, or avoid, sensory experiences. However, children can improve their ability to process sensory information through engagement in appropriate activities and play. This helps to get the level of arousal 'just right'.

Symptoms often displayed by children with sensory integration difficulties, and which may be addressed through the use of a sensory programme, include the following:

- avoidance of touching certain textures, e.g. sticky items

- a need to touch or carry certain objects, e.g. a blanket or soft toy

- sensitivity or abnormal response to light and sounds, e.g. covering eyes or ears

- high activity levels and a tendency to seek out movement, e.g. fidgeting or spinning

- poor concentration and attention to task
- delay in the development of self-care skills, e.g. dressing or feeding
- excessive eye flickering and grimacing
- poor behaviour and non-compliance.

These sensory processing experiences may involve the child being over-aroused or under-aroused:

Over-aroused (too much stimulation, child may withdraw from stimuli)

———————— The 'Just Right' arousal level ————————

Under-aroused (too little stimulation, child may seek out stimuli)

A reduction in the particular stimulation can help bring the children down to their 'just right' level. An increase in the particular stimulation can help bring children up to their 'just right' level.

Listed below are examples of over-arousal and under-arousal sensory reactions which may be observed.

	Over-arousal	**Under-arousal**
Sight	Dislike of bright or flickering lights and visually busy environments	Attracted to light, fascinated with reflections, looks intently at objects or mirrors
Sound	Covers ears, light sleeper, dislikes sudden unexpected or loud noises	Bangs objects, seeks noisy environment, makes loud, rhythmic noises
Smell	Dislikes some smells, e.g. cleaning products, perfume	Smells objects, seeks strong odours, e.g. spicy, citrus
Taste	fussy eater, uses tip of tongue for testing, gags or vomits easily, may prefer pureed foods	Eats anything, seeks strong flavours, mouths, licks non-food objects

Touch	Resists many textures, messy play, personal care, e.g. hair washing, certain clothes	Appears unaware of touch, low reaction to pain, unaware of messiness, e.g. runny nose
Movement	Dislikes being upside down or rough and tumble, intolerant of movement	Seeks out movement, e.g. spinning, rocking, jumping, flapping hands
Body position	Rough with toys, turns whole body to look at something, heavy pencil work	Low muscle tone, weak grip, lacks awareness of body positions

All seven senses identified are addressed within the Fuzzy Buzzy Group.

Encouraging appropriate responses

It is possible to encourage appropriate responses in children with sensory processing difficulties by using therapeutic activities: child-centred treatment sessions carried out in a monitored and safe environment where children can be guided through activities which challenge their ability to respond appropriately to sensory input. Such activities help children experiencing processing difficulties to learn through routine and structure, thus enabling them to learn to organize their sensory systems and to make a successful, appropriate response.

If a child presents as avoiding sensory stimulus, treatment is likely to focus on *reducing* the sensitivity, or abnormal reaction, to sensory inputs such as sound or movement. If a child is showing behaviours which exhibit the need to seek certain sensations such as spinning or hand flapping, these inputs can be provided in a controlled and more 'socially acceptable' manner. It has been found that these strategies can help to decrease the behaviours in other situations.

Behaviour

When a child is upset by exposure to a certain noise or smell an adult may become cross if the child refuses to comply with adult direction or displays what appears to be inappropriate behaviour. A vicious circle can then arise, as adult and child alike may become frustrated and tempers can flare.

What adults frequently do not understand is that the child is not necessarily intentionally behaving badly, but is actually finding it difficult to cope with a particular sensory experience. Therefore, it is important to be aware of the fact that the child may be displaying unwanted behaviours as a result of being unable to process, or correctly interpret, the sensory information being received. Behavioural difficulties and sensory difficulties often go hand-in-hand.

The purpose of the Fuzzy Buzzy Group is to help practitioners and parents to understand and address what it is that the child finds difficult to process. It provides guidelines, strategies and activities to enhance coping mechanisms, while gently introducing the child to different sensory stimuli, in a happy and controlled manner.

Confirmation Letter

Dear   Date:

Thank you for agreeing to your child's participation in the Fuzzy Buzzy Group. We are very pleased to tell you that we can offer your child a place.

The group will run for ____ weeks at: _____

_____

Tel: _____

The dates and times are listed below:

Day:	Location:	Time:
Day:	Location:	Time:
Day:	Location:	Time:
Day:	Location:	Time:
Day:	Location:	Time:
Day:	Location:	Time:
Day:	Location:	Time:
Day:	Location:	Time:

Your child will be exploring many sensory experiences using hands and feet. Please ensure your child is wearing old, loose-fitting clothes.

Your child will be required to bring a teddy bear or similar cuddly 'fuzzy' toy along to each session.

If you would like to contact us before the group starts, please do not hesitate to call. Our phone number is at the bottom of this letter.

Yours sincerely,

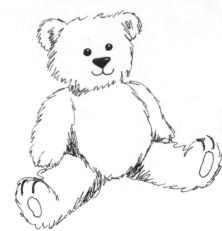

Fuzzy Buzzy Song
(CD track 1)

Fuzzy Buzzy here I come

Fuzzy Buzzy is such fun

I just want to stay and play

Until it's time to go away!

All Together Now
(CD track 2)

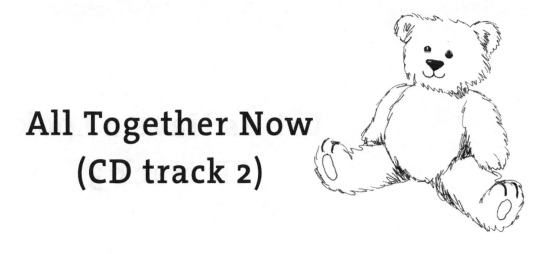

All together now, all together now

Let's all play

All together, all together now

All together now, all together now

Let's all play, all together now!

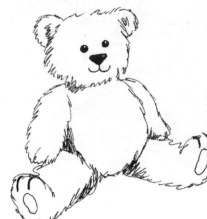

Let Us Have a Look
(CD track 3)

Let us have a look and see

What's inside the bag for me!

Socks and Shoes
(CD track 4)

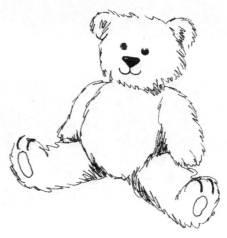

Socks and shoes we'll now take off

Now take off, now take off

Socks and shoes we'll now take off

It is time to take them off

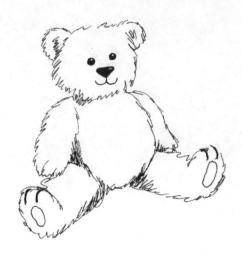

Goodbye
(CD track 5)

Well done, well done

Yes everybody's been very good

You have worked very hard

And been very good

So it's time to say goodbye

Yes it's time to say goodbye

Feeding Checklist

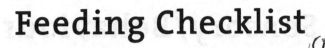

Child's name:		
Date	Food/drink	Child's reaction

Any additional comments:

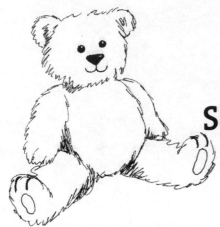

Sensory/Behaviour Form

Child's name:		
Date	**Experience**	**Child's reaction**

Any additional comments:

Evaluation Form

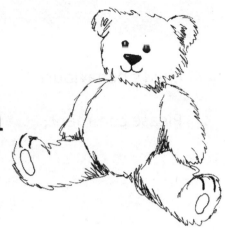

Child's name: _____   **Date:** _____

Please circle **YES** or **NO** where appropriate

Is the child more able to cope in everyday situations?   **YES   NO**

Please comment:

_____

How many of the seven senses is (sight, sound, smell, taste, touch, movement, body position) the child more able to tolerate (if any)?

Please comment:

_____

Have there been improvements observed in the
child's behaviour?   **YES   NO**

Please comment:

_____

Is the child more able to cope with group settings?   **YES   NO**

Please comment:

_____

Are there any improvements in the child's acceptance
of different foods or drink?   **YES   NO**

Please comment:

_____

Do you feel more able to cope with the child's
sensory difficulties as a result of attending the sessions?   **YES   NO**

Please comment:

_____

Do you have a better understanding why the child behaves
the way he/she does?   **YES   NO**

Please comment:

_____

Has the child's social skills improved (e.g. turn-taking,
sharing, waiting, general compliance)?   **YES   NO**

Please comment:

_____

Please use this space to write any further comments you would like to add:

_____

Thank you

Teddy Bear Badge and Sticker Templates

Badges can be photocopied and laminated if desired. Use double-sided sticky tape to stick them to the child's clothes.

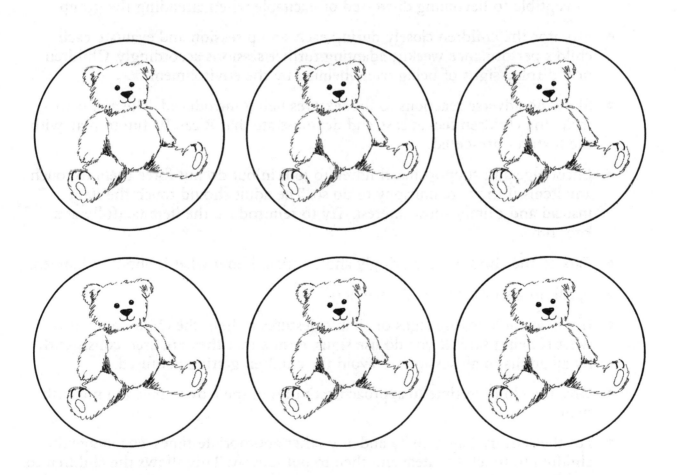

General Tips for Adults Involved in Running a Session

Adults who are involved in the group should work together to plan, deliver and evaluate the activities. They should endeavour to:

- Keep the children calm but interested in the activities. Children may be more susceptible to becoming distressed or excitable when attending the group.

- Monitor the children closely during each group session and evaluate each child's performance weekly, adapting further sessions accordingly. Children may display signs of being overwhelmed by the environment.

- Show no adverse reactions to the textures being introduced. The aim is to make the children feel at ease and demonstrate that it can be fun to play with the textures presented.

- Encourage and support the children to join in but do not force them to touch any items if they are unhappy to do so. The adult should touch the item instead and calmly show interest. Try to reintroduce the item tactfully at a later time.

- Talk to the children reassuringly and let them know what is about to happen.

- Speak in a soothing, gentle manner.

- If you are able to, use signs or simple gestures to help the children focus on what is being said. If you do use signs, ensure that they are used consistently by all adults in all sessions to avoid the children getting confused.

- Give the children time to approach activities in their own time. Do not rush them.

- For the sensory bag activity and any other appropriate times, encourage the children to touch the item and then to put it away. This allows the children to feel in control.

- Walk with the children along the path, hand in hand, in the gross motor 'sensory path' section.

- Always praise any effort made; you can even offer praise at times when the child is not doing anything troublesome, e.g. 'Good sitting!' 'That's nice playing!'

- Finally, make sure you have fun, enjoy the group and build up relationships!

Watching out for over-stimulation

Children may become over-stimulated when engaged in sensory activities. The warning signs can be subtle and may be displayed by a child

- grimacing

- trying to escape

- vocalizing in protest

- becoming frozen or rigid

- generally being upset or crying

- displaying excessive eye flickering or yawning.

Look out for these signs and, if you see them, try to calm and reassure the child.

Fuzzy Buzzy Session Planner

Session number: _____

Duration (approx)	Activity
5 minutes	Hello
10 minutes	Sensory bag containing: _____
10 minutes	Liquidizer flavour: _____
5 minutes	Teddies taken away in pram to hide
10 minutes	Sensory path featuring: _____
15 minutes	Snack time food flavour: _____
5 minutes	Goodbye song

Hand out teddy bear badges or stickers before the children go home.

DATE DUE
